7 EXERCISE FOR SENIORS :
Simple Home Exercises to Boost Confidence, and Boost Energy for Seniors

Bradley S. Harrison

Table of content

Chapter 1

Losing weight with whole body vibration

It's unclear whether whole-body vibration is as healthy for you as regular exercise, although it can provide some fitness and health benefits.

You stand, sit, or lie on a machine with a vibrating platform when you use whole-body vibration. Your body receives energy from the machine's vibrations, which causes your muscles to contract and relax several times every second. You can feel like you're exerting yourself during the activity.

A whole-body vibration machine might be available at your neighborhood gym, or you might buy one to use at home.

Whole-body vibration therapy has been shown to help with weight loss, fat burning, improving flexibility, increasing blood flow, reducing muscular stiffness after exercise, increasing strength, and lowering cortisol levels, according to proponents.

But there is a dearth of a thorough study on whole-body vibration. It's not yet known whether whole-body vibration offers the same variety of health advantages as an exercise that requires active participation, like walking, riding, or swimming.

Whole-body vibration may assist increase muscle strength and aid in weight loss when combined with calorie restriction, according to some research.

Beyond sports and fitness, whole-body vibration might also be useful. According to several studies, when done appropriately and when medical supervision is required, whole-body vibration can:

lower back ache

Improving older adults' strength and balance
minimize bone loss
However, if you want to slim down and get more fit, eat a nutritious diet and get some exercise every day. If you opt for whole-body vibration, don't forget to combine it with cardio and strength training exercises.

Additionally, before utilizing whole-body vibration, especially if you're pregnant or have any health issues, consult with your doctor because it might be detrimental in some circumstances.

Along with conventional equipment, vibration machines have begun to appear in gyms. According to the producers, ten minutes of vibration every day can be comparable to an hour of exercise. Some suggestions standing on a platform that shakes violently may increase blood flow and muscle tone while quickening weight reduction.

The idea of doing nothing while passively standing on a platform while your body appears to tone up and lose weight is intriguing. But is there proof that these vibration machines do what they claim to do?

How does it function?
To increase the efficacy of their training, athletes used whole-body vibration therapy at first. Squats, press-ups, and step-ups, among other common conditioning and gym exercises, would be performed on vibration platforms.

On specially developed equipment that oscillates, typically in a horizontal plane at relatively high frequencies, the therapy is performed while standing, sitting, lying down, or performing exercises.

Receive news that is independent, unbiased, and based on facts.

According to the notion, the vibration signals are carried by body tissues, tendons, and muscles, increasing muscle contractions and enhancing muscle strength, coordination, and balance in the process. Long-term, these contractions would boost muscle hypertroph and energy expenditure, improving blood sugar regulation.

Additionally, according to current research, bone cells are responsive to this vibration and respond by boosting bone density. Better sugar control is a result of this.

However, these remain only theories. Scientific studies use a wide range of vibration parameters, making it difficult to determine the overall effects of whole-body vibration therapy.

In a recent study, whole-body vibration was found to be similar to exercise for improving bone health, blood sugar control, and muscle quality in male mice that were purposely engineered to become obese and diabetic.

Additionally, it was equal in terms of lowering "bad" fat tissue, particularly in the abdomen. However, care should be taken when extrapolating conclusions from this or any other animal study to people.

The results of human trials for whole-body vibration therapy were found to be far less persuasive. Whole-body vibration therapy alone (without exercise) does not assist in significant weight loss. This is often true three times per week, for ten to sixty minutes each day over intervals of six to 52 weeks (considered to be more than 5 percent body weight).

Small-scale individual studies that measure weight loss frequently include diets and other forms of exercise in their methodology. With just whole-body vibration therapy, these advantages are rarely observed.

However, isolated whole-body vibration therapy does increase physical fitness, muscle strength, bone health, and functional capacity to a similar amount as the currently advised 30 to 60 minutes of light to moderate exercise per day when used in similar time doses (30 to 60 minutes).

Overall, if you have the physical capacity, walking for 30 minutes with friends or playing outside for 30 minutes with your family would be significantly healthier for you than spending 30 to 60 minutes standing still while being vibrated.

According to a study, using a vibrator to help you lose weight and strengthen your bones may be just as beneficial as using a treadmill. Before you get too excited, this vibrator is not that kind. It is a vibrating platform that may shake or produce whole-body vibration (WBV). Research in the journal Endocrinology found that spending 20 minutes each day on a vibrating platform for three months reduced belly and liver fat and raised levels of osteocalcin, a protein that strengthens bones. With one caveat: you have to be a mouse. This may be exciting news if you don't want to or are unable to engage in a more demanding exercise like treadmill running. Wait until WBV has been tested on humans more fully if you are a human.

These facts of the study on positive vibrations. Two distinct strains of five-week-old mice were gathered by a research team from Augusta University: normal mice and those with genetic alterations that cause obesity and diabetes. The mice were then subjected to one of three 12-week regimens: sedentary behavior, treadmill running regularly, or regular WBV. WBV appeared to help the mice lose weight and improve their diabetes like treadmill jogging (as measured by glucose and insulin tolerance testing). Yes, it's possible that shaking the mice—which makes their muscles contract and relax and puts stress on their bones—is just as effective as stimulating them to engage in more strenuous exercise.

But before you run out and buy a jackhammer or start sitting on a washing machine, remember that the study only tested one particular form of WBV and did not evaluate any other sorts of vibrations. The issues that exposure to various sorts of vibrations can lead to, such as nausea, weariness, vision abnormalities, tissue damage, and talking as though you're speaking into a fan, were enumerated in this Occupational Health and Safety article by Rob Brauch. Does WBV face these issues? Only 12 weeks was the length of the Augusta University trial, which is perhaps insufficient to investigate the long-term effects of WBV.

WBV has not yet been shown to be able to cause weight loss in humans, and it cannot replace all of the advantages of genuine cardiovascular exercise or active sports. (In general, mix up your exercise routines and sessions because sticking to one exercise or piece of equipment won't yield all the benefits and may even put you in danger for injury.) As a result, wait a while before placing your bets on WBV's ability to effectively cure diabetes and promote weight loss. The evidence that is now available for people is still pretty flimsy.

Chapter 2

Opposite arm and leg raise

Do this exercise gently. Try to maintain your body upright at all times, and don't allow one hip to dip lower than the other.

Start on the floor, on your hands and knees.
Tighten your abdominal muscles.
Raise one leg off the floor and hold it straight out behind you. Be cautious not to let your hip slide down since it will twist your trunk.
Hold for around 6 seconds, then drop your leg and switch to the other leg.
Repeat 8 to 12 times on each leg.
Over time, build up to holding for 10 to 30 seconds each time

If you feel comfortable and confident with your leg up, try extending the opposite arm straight out in front of you at the same moment.

The opposing prone arm and leg raise are done by laying flat on your stomach and lifting one arm off the floor while elevating the opposite leg at the same time. This workout targets muscles of the back, buttocks, hips, and shoulders.

Trapezius

The trapezius is a huge diamond-shaped muscle that covers your upper back. It joins to the bones of your neck and mid-back and runs to the collar bone and scapula. The trapezius pushes your shoulders up and puts your shoulder blades closer together.

Erector Spinae

The erector spinae muscles stretch from your neck to your lower back on each side of your spinal column. These muscles bend and straighten your back and they also assist twist your body.

Deltoids

The deltoids give your shoulders their dome-like form. They contain three parts: The anterior, medial and posterior deltoid.

The deltoids originate at your collar bones and shoulder blades and go to your upper arm bones. They move your arms up and out toward your sides.

Gluteus Maximus
The Gluteus maximus creates the fleshy region of your buttocks. They join the pelvic bone and the sacrum, which is the base of the spine, and go down to the top of your thigh bone. The Gluteus maximus is a hip extensor, which means the muscle straightens your hip.

Quadriceps
Four quadriceps muscles provide the front of your thighs its form. They travel from the top of your leg down to the tendon that keeps your kneecap in place. The quadriceps stretch your knees to straighten your legs.

Hamstrings
Four hamstring muscles constitute the rear of your thigh. They go from the bottom of

the pelvic bone down to the summits of the tibia and fibula, or the lower leg bones. The hamstrings bend your knee and they assist the gluteal muscles to straighten your hip.

Arm and leg balance builds strength and stability in the glutes, hamstrings, core, and shoulder. This exercise also improves coordination.

Get down on the floor with your hands straight and beneath your shoulders. Your knees should be bent to 90 degrees, positioning them precisely under your hips.

Tighten your core and stretch one arm forward so that your shoulder is near to your ear. At the same moment, straighten your opposing leg fully behind you, bringing it to hip height. Return to the beginning posture and repeat with your opposing arm and leg.

Avoid overarching your back at the height of the exercise. Focus on keeping a neutral spine throughout the workout.
Don't allow your hips to move side to side throughout the workout.
As you stretch your leg back make sure you clench your glutes for increased stability.

The Opposite Arm and Leg Raise Exercise is an excellent approach to building and maintaining mobility and stability in your hips, shoulders, and core, for a more efficient golf swing and to assist to avoid injury.

The Opposite Arm and Leg Raise Exercise is part of the Golf Injury Prevention series of unique and dynamic exercises that will help to protect you from pain and injury by increasing strength and stability around your most susceptible regions while improving mobility, balance, and joint function.

Steps

Start on your hands and knees, with your core muscles engaged, your hands squarely under your shoulders, and your shoulders pulled away from the floor.

Simultaneously raise your left arm straight in front of you, and stretch your right leg into the air behind you, until they are both parallel to the ground.

Slowly return to the starting position.

Repeat with your right arm and left leg.

Repeat for the required number of repetitions on each side.

Try not to allow any movement in your torso throughout this workout. Keep your abdominal muscles engaged to stabilize your spine.

You should feel it exercising your shoulders, back, core and hips.

Chapter 3

Head and eyes same direction

The following are seven eye exercises that individuals may choose to attempt for the ailments described above:

1. Digital eye strain may become an issue for persons who need to concentrate on a computer screen all day while working.

This helps relieve digital eye strain. A person has to glance at anything 20 feet away for 20 seconds every 20 minutes when working on a computer.

2. Focus change

The focus shift exercise may also assist with digital eye strain. People should execute this workout while seated.
Hold one finger a couple of inches away from one eye.

Focus the sight on the finger.
Move the finger carefully away from the face.
Focus on an item further away, and then back on the finger.
Bring the finger back closer to the eye.
Focus on an item further away.
Repeat three times.

3. Eye motions
This eye movement exercise also helps with digital eye strain.

Close your eyes.
Slowly move the gaze upward, then downward.
Repeat three times.

Slowly shift the eyes to the left, then to the right.
Repeat three times.

4. Figure 8

The figure 8 exercise might also assist reduce digital eye strain.

Focus on a place on the floor roughly 8 feet distant.
Move the eyeballs in the form of figure 8.
Trace the imaginary figure 8 for 30 seconds, then flip the direction.

5. Pencil pushups

Pencil pushups may assist patients with convergence insufficiency. A doctor could suggest this activity as part of vision rehabilitation.

Hold a pencil at arm's length, located between the eyes.

Look at the pencil and attempt to preserve a single picture of it while gently bringing it nearer the nose.

Move the pencil toward the nose until the pencil is no longer a single picture.
Position the pencil at the nearest position where it is still a single picture.
Repeat 20 times.

6. Brock string
The Brock string exercise helps improve eye coordination.

To execute this practice, a person will need a long thread and several colorful beads. They may execute this activity either sitting or standing.

Secure one end of the string to an immovable item, or another person may hold it.
Hold the other end of the string right below the nose.

Place one bead on the strand.
Look squarely at the bead with both eyes open.
If the eyes are operating properly, a person should see the bead and two strings in the form of an X.

If one eye is closed, one of the threads will vanish, which implies that the eye is suppressing. If the individual sees two beads and two threads, the eyes are not concentrated on the bead.

7. Barrel cards

Barrel cards are an effective exercise for exotropia, which is a kind of strabismus.

Draw three red barrels of increasing sizes on one side of a card.
Repeat in green on the reverse side of the card.

Hold the card towards the nose so that the biggest barrel is furthest away.

Stare at the distant barrel until it forms one picture with both colors and the other two images have multiplied.
Maintain the look for around 5 seconds.
Repeat the exercise with the middle and smallest photographs.

Chapter 4

Pain and inflammation

An analysis published in April 2017 in the Cochrane Database of Systematic Reviews looked at many studies that addressed the impact of physical exercise on chronic pain and found evidence of beneficial benefits overall — with the caveat that additional quality research is required. There's a minimal downside to exercise, the researchers found, and the important advantages of remaining active include increased physical function, decreased severity of pain in joints and other regions, and increases in quality of life.

The CDC recommended persons with RA practice low-impact aerobic activity, such as walking, swimming, or bicycling, three to five times a week, ultimately building up to sessions of 30 to 60 minutes each. Just be sure to chat to your doctor about your fitness intentions before you start.

For those with RA, tiredness may be a huge hurdle to keeping active. Research published in January 2014 in the Israel Medical Association Journal indicated that 40 to 80 percent of persons with RA identify symptoms such as weakness, loss of energy, and exhaustion as the most debilitating element of the condition. Especially when accompanied by joint discomfort, weariness may be a big impediment to exercising frequently.

If this is occurring to you, WebMD advises noting that less activity "results in lower muscular strength and eventually may lead to greater arthritis pain and disability."

In other words, don't use RA as an excuse not to exercise. Instead, use it as your incentive to start acting. Start with these seven expert-recommended workouts for RA.

Walking

It's free, you can perform it practically anyplace, no particular training is required, and it's gentle on weary joints. Walking may help you maintain a healthy weight or reduce weight, resulting in less stress on your joints. In addition, walking may boost your heart health and bone health.

The cardiac benefit of exercise is particularly relevant for those with RA since the illness is known to raise the risk for heart disease.

Swimming

The water is a terrific location to stretch your muscles and calm your joints, so visit the pool for aerobic exercise. Swim laps, or try water walking or a water aerobics class. A study published in March 2017 in the American Journal of Physical Medicine & Rehabilitation found that 16 weeks of water-based exercises in women with RA led to significant improvements in joint and other pain, as well as lowered disease activity when compared with the effectiveness of land-based aerobic exercises.

Swimming helps reduce weight, increase mood, and improve sleep, and it's beneficial for general health, says Madhoun.

Strength Training

For those with RA, some joint pain triggers might make symptoms worse. But the stronger your muscles are, the less tension there is on your joints. So don't be frightened of weights, since they're a terrific method to grow stronger and build muscle mass.

Research published in April 2018 in the journal Arthritis Care & Research indicated that in older persons with RA, aerobic and resistance activities combined may enhance aerobic capacity, endurance, and strength.

Experiment with weight machines, free weights, and resistance bands. Start softly and raise your intensity progressively. Aim for two or three days a week, practicing eight to 10 different exercises that engage various main muscle groups throughout your body. Do two or three sets of eight to 12 repetitions of each exercise. Of course, if you experience discomfort, back off a bit.

Cycling

Cycling is a terrific kind of cardiovascular exercise that's gentle on the joints. But it does come with the danger of falling, so it's crucial to purchase the correct sort of bike for your physique. The Arthritis Foundation suggests looking at comfort bikes (cruisers), recumbent cycles, mountain bikes, or hybrid bikes, all of which have excellent stability and handling.

Yoga and Tai Chi

"When a joint and its surrounding muscles are compromised by arthritis, the outcome is typically decreased coordination, position awareness, [and] balance and an increased risk of falling, which is why many complain of their 'knees giving out' with activity," Madhoun explains. He notes that yoga and tai chi are examples of workouts that develop body awareness, which may boost coordination and balance, a feeling of where joints are positioned (proprioception), and relaxation. Plus, they incorporate flexibility and range-of-motion routines, which increase joint flexibility and function, according to the CDC.

Pilates

Pilates focuses on strengthening and developing control of muscles, providing you with a low-impact exercise that may reduce strain on your hips and other joints. Pilates may also be beneficial in controlling pain and dealing with the symptoms of RA. The Arthritis Foundation urges individuals to stay to their speed in a Pilates class and ask the teacher about adaptations if RA symptoms are hurting them.

Balance exercises such as walking backward or standing on one foot are also beneficial for strengthening balance and preventing falls. Just be aware that you may need to adjust certain positions to decrease stress on joints and maybe include props to aid with your balance.

Get Fit at Home

You don't necessarily have to go to the gym or even the streets for decent exercise. There are many things you may do around your house. Give your home a thorough cleaning or work in your yard, removing weeds, raking leaves, or trimming the lawn. While you're at home, practice balancing on one leg to increase strength and balance. Improvise strengthening exercises by utilizing a chair to go from sitting to standing, or hoist hand weights — soup cans can be an excellent replacement! — for some light strength training. For more ideas, talk to a physical therapist or your doctor.

Adjusting Exercise for Your RA

No matter what exercise you undertake with RA, be careful to respect and protect your body with appropriate changes to equipment and varied forms of activity. "When clients are in a flare of their condition, I frequently urge them to concentrate on flexibility and low-impact workouts, such as swimming, yoga, and walking," says Anisha Dua, MD, MPH, a rheumatologist and associate professor at Northwestern Medicine Feinberg School of Medicine in Chicago. "When RA is properly managed, it's tremendously useful to participate in regularly planned physical activity, including aerobic and strengthening exercises." Just remember to complete them with the appropriate posture and form, and allow yourself time to work out.

Mobility is crucial

When you experience inflammatory arthritis pain, it might be tempting to feel like you should move less. But in reality, the reverse is typically true: modest motions, building up to more regular activity, may have a therapeutic impact by lessening the pain and suffering of inflammatory arthritis. When you sit for lengthy durations, your joints might get stiff, and chronic inactivity may even contribute to muscular atrophy.

Incorporating regular physical exercise into your life is crucial when you have inflammatory arthritis. Ideally, your fitness program should include stretching activities to support mobility and decrease stiffness, strengthening exercises to protect and stabilize your joints, and cardiovascular activity to support your heart and enhance the flow of oxygen-rich blood to all areas of your body.

If you're not currently involved in a regular fitness program and want to know where to begin, have a chat with your general care physician or rheumatologist, who may suggest that you visit a physical therapist to discover the best activities for your kind of arthritis. If your arthritis is affecting your hands, wrists, elbows, or shoulders, you may also consider seeing an occupational therapist or certified hand therapist, who is specially trained to focus on the upper extremities of the body – such as exercises for rheumatoid arthritis affecting the hands and fingers.

Which workouts are best for inflammatory arthritis?
While one exercise plan might not work for every person with inflammatory arthritis, here are some activities that many individuals like and find useful for reducing their symptoms. See a physical or occupational therapist learn how to conduct

these things effectively while keeping excellent alignment and posture.

Strengthening exercises
There's no need to rush out and join a gym. You can begin getting stronger at home

Start with sitting to standing exercises, rising from a chair utilizing the muscles of your legs, and then sitting down again.
For the upper body, you may begin by lifting cans of soup or light dumbbells (two to five pounds apiece is acceptable) (two to five pounds each is sufficient).
Some individuals appreciate the resistance treatment supplied by elastic workout bands.

Pilates is good for strengthening your core, which supports the rest of your body.
Stretching exercises

Yoga is a terrific approach to learning gentle stretching of all regions of the body while also strengthening your muscles. Chair yoga is a safe method to perform if you are worried about balance concerns or other constraints. Yin yoga is a peaceful, slow-moving kind of yoga that focuses on maintaining particular postures for three minutes or longer.

Walking.
Hiking, utilizing poles for support and balance as required.
Swimming and water activities, ease the effects of gravity on the joints while delivering light resistance.
T'ai chi is a sequence of gradual, slow motions that enhance mobility as well as balance. Many individuals dealing with arthritis find it to be quite beneficial.

Schedule pauses throughout your day for rest if you are active, and for movement if you are largely sedentary. For example, if you are sitting at a computer for many hours, make little body movements every 15 to 20 minutes, such as extending your hands, arms, and neck in your chair. Every 45 minutes, get up to move the bigger joints of your body, such as using the toilet or grabbing a drink of water.

"No suffering" does not equal "no gain"
There is a myth that exercise has to induce pain or suffering for you to realize that it's working. But this is not always true. If you continue to undertake the sorts of activities that assist persons with inflammatory arthritis, you will experience gains in various ways: less pain, improved function, less energy needed to move, and more mobility.

Aligning with a physical or occupational therapist who knows your needs and preferences may help you develop objectives that work for you. You don't need to go to therapy sessions forever; even just two to three sessions to put together a movement plan for you can have lasting benefits. Occupational therapists may also fit clients with personalized splints or pair them with adaptive equipment to make it simpler and more pleasant to go through the day.

Restoring energy flow: acupuncture for inflammatory arthritis

Many patients have claimed improvement in their symptoms after undergoing acupuncture for rheumatoid arthritis, psoriatic arthritis, and other kinds of inflammatory arthritis. Acupuncture includes the insertion of extremely thin needles into critical spots in the body, to restore the flow of energy, or "qi."

Note that the acupuncture energy points for arthritis may not be in the same region where you may be experiencing pain, and that's good; a qualified acupuncturist understands where to enter the needles to get the maximum benefit to match your requirements. Acupuncture has also been demonstrated to help ease muscular tension, reduce stress, and promote better sleep. "Tui na" massage treatment is a comparable ancient Chinese method that stimulates particular acupressure sites without needles. Both treatments tend to have the greatest effect when your inflammation is not at its highest (such as during a flare), but rather after your symptoms have settled a little.

The mind is the master
Meditation and psychotherapy (especially cognitive-behavioral or "talk" therapy) has

benefited many patients with inflammatory arthritis by addressing the worry and stress that may increase symptoms. Cognitive-behavioral therapy may help you redefine your connection with your arthritis symptoms so you don't let them overwhelm your thinking.

Meditation and measured breathing have been demonstrated to lower stress and the consequences of inflammation by stimulating your vagus nerve, which helps you react better to stress. Try repeating this method eight times, twice a day:

Breathe deep into your abdomen for four counts.
Hold for seven counts.
Exhale for eight counts.
It might be tempting to let severe, chronic arthritic symptoms steal the fun out of life, but you don't have to. With coaching from

certified specialists, you may begin moving again and use mind-body practices that enable you to manage your pain, rather than having it dominate you.